ANTI INFLAMMATORY DIET COOKBOOK

DR. PENNY WATSON

Copyright © 2023 by Dr. Penny Watson

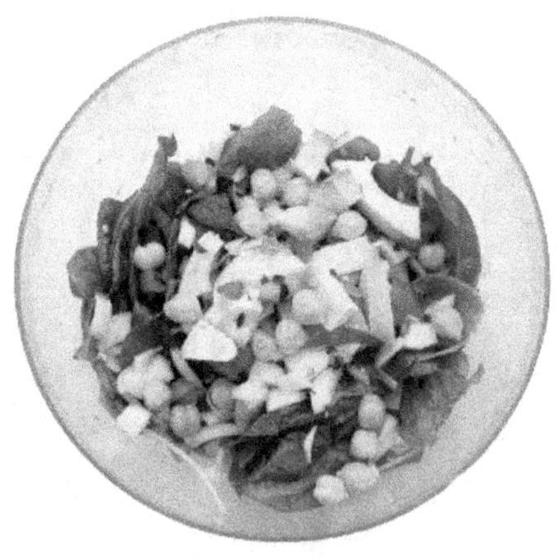

TABLE OF CONTENTS

INTRODUCTION

Inflammation is your body's way of protecting itself from infection, illness, or injury. As part of the inflammatory response, your body increases its production of white blood cells, immune cells, and substances called cytokines that help fight infection.

Classic signs of acute (short-term) inflammation include redness, pain, heat, and swelling. On the other hand, chronic (long-term) inflammation often occurs inside your body without any noticeable symptoms. This type of inflammation can drive illnesses like diabetes, heart disease, fatty liver disease, and cancer. Chronic inflammation can also happen when people are obese or under stress. When doctors look for inflammation, they test for a few markers in your blood, including C-reactive protein (CRP), homocysteine, TNF alpha, and IL-6.

What Causes Inflammation

Certain lifestyle factors — especially habitual ones — can promote inflammation. Consuming high amounts of sugar and high-fructose corn syrup is particularly harmful.

It can lead to insulin resistance, diabetes, and obesity. Scientists have also hypothesized that consuming a lot of refined carbs, such as white bread, may contribute to inflammation, insulin resistance, and obesity. What's more, eating processed and packaged foods that contain trans fats has been shown to promote inflammation and damage the endothelial cells that line your arteries. Vegetable oils used in many processed foods are another possible culprit. Regular consumption may result in an imbalance of omega-6 to omega-3 fatty acids, which some scientists believe may promote inflammation. Excessive intake of alcohol and processed meat can also have inflammatory effects on your body. Additionally, an inactive lifestyle that includes a lot of sitting is a major non-dietary factor that can promote inflammation.

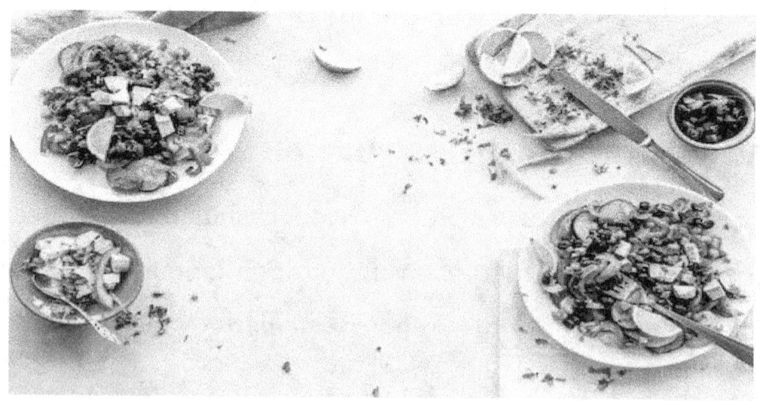

CHAPTER ONE

The Role of Your Diet In Treating Inflammation

If you want to reduce inflammation, eat fewer inflammatory foods and more anti-inflammatory foods. Base your diet on whole, nutrient-dense foods that contain antioxidants — and avoid processed products. Antioxidants work by reducing levels of free radicals.

These reactive molecules are created as a natural part of your metabolism but can lead to inflammation when they're not held in check.

Your anti-inflammatory diet should provide a healthy balance of protein, carbs, and fat at each meal.

Make sure you also meet your body's needs for vitamins, minerals, fiber, and water.

One diet considered anti-inflammatory is the Mediterranean diet, which has been shown to reduce inflammatory markers, such as CRP and IL-6.

A low-carb diet also reduces inflammation, particularly for people who are obese or have metabolic syndrome.

In addition, vegetarian diets are linked to reduced inflammation.

Anti-inflammatory diet What to know

Inflammation helps the body fight illness and can protect it from harm. In most cases, it is a necessary part of the healing process.

However, some people have a medical condition in which the immune system does not work as it should. This malfunction can lead to persistent or recurrent low level inflammation. Chronic inflammation occurs with various diseases, such as psoriasis, rheumatoid arthritis, and asthma.

There is evidence that dietary choices may help manage the symptoms. An anti-inflammatory diet favors fruits and vegetables, foods containing omega-3 fatty acids, whole grains, lean protein, healthful fats, and spices. It discourages or limits the consumption of processed foods, red meats, and alcohol. The anti-inflammatory diet is not a specific regimen but rather a style of eating.

The Mediterranean diet and the DASH diet are examples of anti-inflammatory diets.

What Is an Anti-Inflammatory Diet?

Share on PinterestThe anti-inflammatory diet includes nutrient-dense plant foods and avoids processed foods and meats. Some foods contain ingredients that can trigger or worsen inflammation. Sugary or processed foods may do this, while fresh, whole foods are less likely to have this effect.

An anti-inflammatory diet focuses on fresh fruits and vegetables. Many plant-based foods are good sources of antioxidants. Some foods, however, can trigger the formation of free radicals. Examples include foods that people fry in repeatedly heated cooking oil.

Dietary antioxidants are molecules in food that help remove free radicals from the body. Free radicals are the natural byproducts of some bodily processes, including metabolism. However, external factors, such as stress and smoking, can increase the number of free radicals in the body. Free radicals can lead to cell damage. This damage increases the risk of inflammation and can contribute to a range of diseases. The body creates some antioxidants that help it removes these toxic substances, but dietary antioxidants also help.

An anti-inflammatory diet favors foods that are rich in antioxidants over those that increase the production of free radicals. Omega-3 fatty acids, which are present in oily fish, may help reduce the levels of inflammatory proteins in the body. Fiber can also have this effect, according to the Arthritis Foundation.

Types of Anti-Inflammatory diet

Many popular diets already adhere to anti-inflammatory principles.

For example, both the Mediterranean diet and the DASH diet include fresh fruits and vegetables, fish, whole grains, and fats that are good for the heart.

Inflammation appears to play a role in cardiovascular disease, but research suggests that the Mediterranean diet, with its focus on plant-based foods and healthful oils, can reduce the effects of inflammation on the cardiovascular system.

Who can it help?

An anti-inflammatory diet may serve as a complementary therapy for many conditions that become worse with chronic inflammation.

The following conditions involve inflammation:

• rheumatoid arthritis

• psoriasis

• asthma

• eosinophilic esophagitis

• Crohn's disease

• colitis

• inflammatory bowel disease

• lupus

• Hashimoto's thyroiditis

• metabolic syndrome

Metabolic syndrome refers to a collection of conditions that tend to occur together, including type 2 diabetes, obesity, high blood pressure, and cardiovascular disease. Scientists believe that inflammation plays a role in all of these. An anti-inflammatory diet may, therefore, help improve the health of a person with metabolic syndrome.

Eating a diet that is rich in antioxidants may also help reduce the risk of certain cancers.

Foods to eat on an Anti-Inflammatory Diet

An anti-inflammatory diet should combine a variety of foods that:

• Are rich in nutrients

• Provide a range of antioxidants

• Contain healthful fats

Foods that may help manage inflammation include:

• Oily fish, such as tuna and salmon

• Fruits, such as blueberries, blackberries, strawberries, and cherries

• Vegetables, including kale, spinach, and broccoli

• Beans

• Nuts and seeds

• Olives and olive oil

• Fiber

The authors of a 2017 article also recommended the following:

• Raw or moderately cooked vegetables

• Legumes, such as lentils

• Spices, such as ginger and turmeric

• Probiotics and prebiotics

• Tea

• Some herbs

It is worth remembering that: No single food will boost a person's health. It is important to include a variety of healthful ingredients in the diet.

Fresh, simple ingredients are best. Processing can change the nutritional content of foods.

People should check the labels of premade foods. While cocoa can be a good choice, for example, the products that contain cocoa often also contain sugar and fat.

A colorful plate will provide a range of antioxidants and other nutrients.

Be sure to vary the colors of fruits and vegetables.

Foods to avoid on Anti-Inflammatory Diet

People who are following an anti-inflammatory diet should avoid or limit their intake of:

• Processed foods

• Foods with added sugar or salt

• Unhealthful oils

• Processed carbs, which are present in white bread, white pasta, and many baked goods

• Processed snack foods, such as chips and crackers

• Premade desserts, such as cookies, candy, and ice cream

• Excess alcohol

• In addition, people may find it beneficial to limit their intake of the following:

Gluten: Some people experience an inflammatory reaction when they consume gluten. A gluten-free diet can be restrictive, and it is not suitable for everyone. However, if a person suspects that gluten is triggering symptoms, they may wish to consider eliminating it for a while to see if their symptoms improve.

Nightshades: Plants belonging to the nightshade family, such as tomatoes, eggplants, peppers, and potatoes, seem to trigger flares in some people with inflammatory diseases.

There is limited evidence to confirm this effect, but a person can try cutting nightshades from the diet for 2–3 weeks to see if their symptoms improve.

Carbohydrates: There is some evidence that a high carb diet, even when the carbs are healthful, may promote inflammation in some people.

However, some carb-rich foods, such as sweet potatoes and whole grains, are excellent sources of antioxidants and other nutrients.

Can a vegetarian diet reduce inflammation?

A vegetarian diet may be one option for people looking to reduce inflammation. The authors of a 2019 review analyzed data from 40 studies. They concluded that people who follow a vegetarian-based diet are likely to have lower levels of various inflammatory markers.

A 2017 study looked at the data of 268 people who followed either a strict vegetarian diet, a lacto-ovo-vegetarian diet, or a nonvegetarian diet. The findings suggested that eating animal products could increase the risk of systemic inflammation and insulin resistance. Earlier research from 2014 suggested that lower inflammation levels could be a key benefit of a vegan diet.

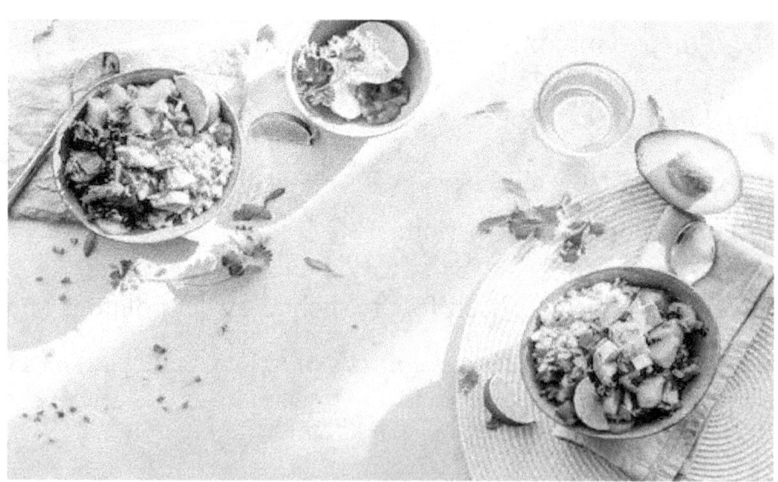

CHAPTER TWO

Anti-inflammatory Diet Tips

It can be challenging to transition to a new way of eating, but the following tips may help:

• Pick up a variety of fruits, vegetables, and healthful snacks during the weekly shop.

• Gradually replace fast food meals with healthful, homemade lunches.

• Replace soda and other sugary beverages with still or sparkling mineral water.

Other tips include

• Talking to a healthcare professional about supplements, such as cod liver oil or a multivitamin.

• Incorporating 30 minutes of moderate exercise into the daily routine.

• Practicing good sleep hygiene, as poor sleep can worsens inflammation.

One-Day Sample Menu

It's easier to stick to a diet when you have a plan. Here's a great sample menu to start you out, featuring a day of anti-inflammatory meals:

Breakfast

• 3-egg omelet with 1 cup (110 grams) of mushrooms and 1 cup (67 grams) of kale, cooked in olive oil

• 1 cup (225 grams) of cherries

• Green tea and/or water

Lunch

• Grilled salmon on a bed of mixed greens with olive oil and vinegar

• 1 cup (125 grams) of raspberries, topped with plain Greek yogurt and chopped pecans

• Unsweetened iced tea, water

Snack

• Bell pepper strips with guacamole

Dinner

• Chicken curry with sweet potatoes, cauliflower, and broccoli

• Red wine (5–10 ounces or 140–280 ml)

• 1 ounce (30 grams) of dark chocolate (preferably at least 80% cocoa).

Other Helpful Tips

Once you have your healthy menu organized, make sure you incorporate these other good habits of an anti-inflammatory lifestyle:

• Supplements: Certain supplements can reduce inflammation, including fish oil and curcumin.

• Regular exercise: Exercise can decrease inflammatory markers and your risk of chronic disease.

• Sleep: Getting enough sleep is extremely important. Researchers have found that a poor night's sleep increases inflammation.

TYPES OF ANTI-INFLAMMATORY DIETS

Long before the invention of cheese curls, chicken nuggets, soda and all the other ultra-processed foods that make up the bulk of the average American diet, people around the globe thrived on their traditional diets.

As different as a Chinese stir-fry might seem from a fresh Italian pasta topped with marinara sauce, at its core, a traditional diet meets an anti-inflammatory diet checklist.

Below is a roundup of the more well-researched anti-inflammatory eating patterns from across the world, as well as the DASH diet, which takes its cue from traditional diets.

Traditional Mediterranean Diet

Italy, Greece, the south of France, Lebanon and other countries along the Mediterranean Sea have unique cuisines, but they share many of the same ingredients.

Research suggests the Mediterranean diet helps ward off a bevy of inflammatory-based diseases, including obesity, cardiovascular diseases, stroke, type 2 diabetes, certain cancers, allergies, Parkinson's disease and Alzheimer's disease.

To pluck just one study of hundreds, researchers tracked thousands of Greek adults ages 20 to 86 for four years. For those adhering most closely to a Mediterranean-style diet, deaths from heart disease dropped by one-third, and the group experienced a quarter fewer cancer deaths and deaths from any cause.

Characteristics of a traditional Mediterranean diet include:

• A wide diversity of fruit, vegetables and minimally processed grains and legumes form the bulk of the diet.

• Olive oil, nuts and seeds are the main fat sources.

• Fish is the principal animal protein. A small portion of red meat is eaten just once every week or two.

• Small amounts of cheese and yogurt are the principal dairy foods, with next to no butter or cream.

• Wine is allowed in low to moderate amounts and only with meals.

• Sweets are relegated to celebrations and based on nuts, olive oil and honey.

A favorite snack: figs stuffed with walnuts.

Traditional Okinawan Diet

Okinawa is a Japanese island famous for having a high rate of its people reach 100 years old in good health. The local diet gets much of the credit.

The overall dietary pattern is dominated by anti-inflammatory vegetables, particularly Okinawan sweet potatoes," says Bradley J. Willcox, M.D., a professor of geriatric medicine and director of research at the Department of Geriatric Medicine for the John A. Burns School of Medicine at the University of Hawaii.

"They also have the highest soy consumption in Japan, and likely, the world," he says, adding the diet also boasts low amounts of pro-inflammatory foods, such as added sugar, saturated fat and red meat.

A traditional Okinawan diet is:

• Low calorie

• Rich in vegetables, including seaweed

• Rich in legumes, particularly soy

• Moderate in fish

• Low in meat and dairy

• Moderate in alcohol

While this may sound like any other healthy diet, there are unique elements, such as:

• It contains lots of soy. The diet averages about 3 ounces of tofu, miso and other soy foods daily. Soy contains anti-inflammatory isoflavones and other protective compounds, and is linked to cardiovascular health.

• It's rich in seaweed. You may be familiar with nori—the dark sushi wrapper— but it's just one of more than a dozen types of seaweed in Okinawan cuisine. They're rich in protective compounds, such as astaxanthin, a powerful antioxidant and inflammation-quencher.

• Okinawan sweet potato is the main starch. Sure, it's eaten in other cuisines, but it's not fried and is the main starch in the traditional Okinawan diet.

It's rich in anti-inflammatory nutrients such as beta-carotene (the orange pigment), anthocyanins and vitamins E and C.

• It's low-fat. The Okinawan diet certainly shares similarities with the popular Mediterranean diet, but its main differentiator is that it has far less fat, says Willcox. While the Mediterranean diet typically consists of 30% to 40% healthy, mainly monounsaturated fats, the traditional Okinawan diet consists of only about 10% fat.

Traditional Nordic Diet

The cuisines of Denmark, Sweden and Finland differ, but traditionally, they share core healthy foods, including:

• Whole rye products (bread, muesli)

• Berries

• Apples

• Pears

• Fish

• Cabbage

• Broccoli

• Sauerkraut

• Carrots

• Potatoes

• Canola oil as the principle oil

These foods provide anti-inflammatory benefits due to a wealth of nutrients. Rye deserves a special shoutout—it's a grain that's been shown to help reduce blood sugar, the inflammatory marker C-reactive protein, and PSA (a marker for prostate cancer in men).

People who adhere more closely to this way of eating have lower blood levels of C-reactive protein and other markers of inflammation, according to a University of Eastern Finland review of the research.

Especially protective are fruit (apples, pears, berries), grains (rye, oat and barley) and diets that limit non-lean and processed meat and keep alcohol in moderation.

The review also found that even a short-term stint on a healthy Nordic diet can improve certain inflammatory markers and trim off pounds. The randomized studies—done in various Nordic countries, and lasting six to 24 weeks—assigned a healthy Nordic diet to one group while the other stayed on the modern (and less healthy) diet of the country.

A healthy Nordic diet may also have big payoffs when it comes to type 2 diabetes protection, a disease closely linked with chronic inflammation. In a study tracking 57,053 middle-aged Danes for 15 years, those whose diet most closely mirrored a healthy Nordic pattern cut risk for type 2 diabetes by 25% (for women) and 38% (for men), compared to people whose diets strayed most from the healthy paradigm.

Traditional Mexican Diet

Another popular, anti-inflammatory eating pattern hails from Mexico. Mainstays of a traditional Mexican diet include:

• Corn tortillas

• Beans

• A wealth of fruits and vegetables (including hot peppers)

• Rice (brown and white)

• Cheese

Indeed, research has linked a traditional Mexican diet to lower inflammation. A National Cancer Institute-funded study of 493 post-menopausal women of Mexican descent living in the U.S. found that those following a more traditional Mexican diet averaged a 23% lower CRP score—the blood marker of inflammation.

Legumes, which play a starring role in Mexican cuisine, are linked to protection from an impressive lineup of inflammatory-related conditions: High blood pressure, obesity, high blood cholesterol, type 2 diabetes and cardiovascular disease. How does a bean-based diet manage all that? According to a review in Advances in Nutrition much of the credit goes to its very high fiber level, which has bodywide effects:

• Reduces inflammation, especially when legumes replace red meat

• Reduces "bad" cholesterol

• Blunts the rise in blood sugar after a meal, which over time helps prevent type 2 diabetes and inflammation

• Quells appetite, which helps with weight loss

Legumes are so nutritious that the Dietary Guidelines for Americans recommends we consume them weekly.

Dietary Approaches to Stop Hypertension (DASH)

The DASH diet was created in the 1990s in the United States as a way to lower high blood pressure (hypertension).

It does that—and more. A 2018 review of several studies found that DASH significantly lowers CRP compared to a typical American diet.

DASH follows the anti-inflammation playbook.

It's rich in fruits and vegetables, most grains are whole, its protein sources are mainly fish, poultry and legumes and it limits pro-inflammatory foods such as red meat, sweets and sugary beverages.

Another perk of the DASH Diet is that it can lower your LDL. Excessive saturated fat raises LDL—the "bad" blood cholesterol—but DASH limits foods high in this fat, which are also known to trigger inflammation.

These foods include fatty meat, high-fat dairy (butter, cream, cheese, whole milk), and coconut, palm and palm kernel oils. Instead, the menu features fat-free or low-fat dairy and vegetable oils, such as canola, corn, olive and safflower oil.

ANTI-INFLAMMATORY DIET TIPS

1. Consume at least 25 grams of fiber every day

A fiber-rich diet can help reduce inflammation by supplying naturally occurring anti-inflammatory phytonutrients found in fruits, vegetables, and other whole foods. To get your fill of fiber, seek out whole grains, fruits, and vegetables. The best sources include whole grains such as barley and oatmeal; vegetables like okra, eggplant, and onions; and a variety of fruits like bananas (3 grams of fiber per banana) and blueberries (3.5 grams of fiber per cup).

2. Eat a minimum of nine servings of fruits and vegetables every day

One "serving" is half a cup of a cooked fruit or vegetable, or one cup of a raw leafy vegetable. For an extra punch, add anti-inflammatory herbs and spices—such as turmeric and ginger—to your cooked fruits and vegetables to increase the benefits.

3. Eat four servings of both alliums and crucifers every week

Alliums include garlic, scallions, onions, and leek, while crucifers refer to vegetables such as broccoli, cabbage, cauliflower, mustard greens, and Brussels sprouts. Because of their powerful antioxidant properties, consuming a weekly average of four servings of each can help lower your risk of cancer. If you like the taste, I recommend eating a clove of garlic a day.

4. Limit saturated fat to 10 percent of your daily calories

By keeping saturated fat low (that's about 20 grams per 2,000 calories), you'll help reduce the risk of heart disease. You should also limit red meat to once per week and marinate it with herbs, spices, and tart, unsweetened fruit juices to reduce the toxic compounds formed during cooking.

5. Consume foods rich in omega-3 fatty acids

Research suggests that omega-3 fatty acids reduce inflammation and may help lower risk of chronic diseases such as heart disease, cancer, and arthritis conditions that often have a high inflammatory process at their root.

Aim to eat lots of foods high in omega-3 fatty acids like flax meal, walnuts, and beans such as navy, kidney and soy. I also recommend taking a good-quality omega-3 supplement.

6. Eat fish at least three times a week

Fish are another fantastic omega-3 rich food. Go for cold-water fish such as salmon, oysters, herring, mackerel, trout, sardines, and anchovies.

Low-fat fish such as sole and flounder, may also have anti-inflammatory benefits.

7. Use oils that contain healthy fats

The body requires fat, but choose the fats that provide you with benefits. Virgin and extra-virgin olive oil (organic if possible) are the best bets for anti-inflammatory benefits. Other options include high-oleic, expeller-pressed versions of sunflower and safflower oil.

8. Eat healthy snacks twice a day

If you're a snacker, aim for fruit, plain or unsweetened Greek-style yogurt (it contains more protein per serving), celery sticks, carrots, or nuts like pistachios, almonds, and walnuts.

9. Avoid processed foods and refined sugars

This includes any food that contains high-fructose corn syrup or is high in sodium, which contribute to inflammation throughout the body. Avoid refined sugars whenever possible and artificial sweeteners altogether. The dangers of excess fructose have been widely cited and include increased insulin resistance (which can lead to type-2 diabetes), raised uric acid levels, raised blood pressure, increased risk of fatty liver disease, and more.

10. Cut out trans fats

In 2006, the FDA required food manufacturers to identify trans fats on nutrition labels, and for good reason—studies suggest that people who eat foods high in trans fats have higher levels of C-reactive protein, a biomarker for inflammation in the body.

A good rule of thumb is to always read labels and steer clear of products that contain the words "hydrogenated" or "partially hydrogenated oils." Vegetable shortenings, select margarines, crackers, and cookies are just a few examples of foods that might contain trans fats.

11. Sweeten meals with phytonutrient-rich fruits, and flavor foods with spices

Most fruits and vegetables are loaded with important phytonutrients. In order to naturally sweeten your meals, try adding apples, apricots, berries, and even carrots. And for flavoring savory meals, go for spices that are known for their anti-inflammatory properties, including cloves, cinnamon, turmeric, rosemary, ginger, sage, and thyme.

How to Follow Anti Inflammatory Diet

Following an anti-inflammatory diet can have numerous health benefits. Here's a step-by-step guide on how to follow an anti-inflammatory diet:

1. Understand the Basics:

Educate yourself about inflammation and its connection to various health issues. Chronic inflammation has been linked to conditions like heart disease, diabetes, arthritis, and more. Learn about foods that promote inflammation (such as sugary and processed foods) and those that have anti-inflammatory properties (like fruits, vegetables, and certain fats).

2. Prioritize Whole Foods:

Focus on whole, unprocessed foods. Choose fresh fruits, vegetables, whole grains, lean proteins, and healthy fats. Minimize or avoid processed foods, sugary snacks, fast food, and foods with high levels of trans fats and saturated fats.

3. Embrace Colorful Produce:

Incorporate a variety of colorful fruits and vegetables into your meals. These foods are rich in antioxidants and phytochemicals that can help combat inflammation.

Aim for a wide range of colors to ensure you're getting a diverse array of nutrients.

4. Include Omega-3 Fatty Acids:

Consume sources of omega-3 fatty acids, such as fatty fish (salmon, mackerel, sardines), walnuts, flaxseeds, and chia seeds. Omega-3s have potent anti-inflammatory properties.

5. Opt for Healthy Fats:

Choose healthy fats like olive oil, avocados, and nuts. These fats contain compounds that can help reduce inflammation.

6. Limit Processed Meats and Red Meat:

Minimize consumption of processed meats (like sausages and bacon) and red meat. These meats have been associated with increased inflammation.

7. Incorporate Lean Proteins:

Opt for lean protein sources, such as poultry, fish, legumes (beans, lentils, chickpeas), and tofu.

8. Choose Whole Grains:

Replace refined grains (white bread, white rice) with whole grains (brown rice, quinoa, whole wheat). Whole grains have more fiber and nutrients that can help reduce inflammation.

9. Spices and Herbs:

Include anti-inflammatory spices and herbs in your cooking, such as turmeric, ginger, garlic, and cinnamon. These ingredients have natural anti-inflammatory properties.

10. Reduce Added Sugars:

Minimize consumption of sugary beverages, desserts, and processed snacks. Excess sugar intake can contribute to inflammation.

11. Hydration:

Drink plenty of water throughout the day to stay hydrated. Water supports bodily functions and can help flush out toxins.

12. Plan Balanced Meals:

Create balanced meals that include a combination of lean protein, healthy fats, fiber-rich carbohydrates, and a variety of vegetables.

13. Be Mindful of Portion Sizes:

Practice portion control to avoid overeating, which can contribute to weight gain and inflammation.

14. Consult a Professional:

If you have specific health concerns or medical conditions, consider consulting a registered dietitian, nutritionist, or healthcare provider before making significant dietary changes.

Remember that adopting an anti-inflammatory diet is a lifestyle change, and consistency is key.

CHAPTER THREE

Delicous Anti-Inflammatory Diet Recipes

1. Chickpea Shawarma Salad

INGREDIENTS

• 1 15-ounce can chickpeas (rinsed, drained and dried in a clean towel)

• 1 Tbsp olive oil

• 1 heaping tsp cumin

• 1/2 heaping tsp smoked paprika

• 1/2 heaping tsp turmeric

• 1/2 scant tsp sea salt

• 1/2 tsp ground cinnamon

• 1/4 tsp ground ginger

• 1 pinch each black pepper, ground coriander + cardamom

• 5 ounces spring mix lettuce (organic when possible)

• 10 cherry tomatoes (chopped // organic when possible)

• 1/4 cup red onion (thinly sliced)

• 3/4 cup fresh parsley

• 20 pita chips (slightly crushed // store-bought or homemade // gluten-free if GF, or sub gluten-free crackers or cooked quinoa)

DRESSING

• 1/2 cup hummus (DIY or store-bought)

• 3 cloves garlic (3 cloves yield ~ 1 1/2 Tbsp // finely minced or grated)

• 1 tsp dried dill (or sub 2 tsp fresh dill per 1 tsp dried)

• 1 medium lemon, juiced (1 lemon yields ~2 Tbsp or 30 ml)

• Water (to thin)

INSTRUCTIONS

1. Preheat oven to 400 degrees F (204 C) and position a rack in the middle of the oven.

2. Add washed and dried chickpeas to a mixing bowl. Add olive oil and all seasoning and toss to combine. To help them cook faster and disperse the seasonings more easily, lightly

mash half the chickpeas with a fork (leaving the other half whole).

3. Sample a chickpea and adjust seasonings as needed (I added more salt, cumin, and ginger). Then arrange in a single layer on a bare baking sheet and bake for 20-22 minutes, or until golden brown and crispy. Then set aside.

4. In the meantime, prepare all salad ingredients and add to a bowl (reserving pita chips for later). Set aside.

5. To prepare dressing, add hummus, garlic, dill, and lemon juice to a small mixing bowl and whisk to combine. Then add warm water and whisk until pourable.

6. To serve, add baked chickpeas and pita chips to the salad, along with half of the dressing. Toss to combine.

7. Divide between serving dishes and serve with remaining dressing.

8. For best results, store leftovers separately (chickpeas in a container at room temperature, salad ingredients in refrigerator, dressing in a container in refrigerator, pita chips in a container at room temperature). Keeps for 2-3 days, though best when fresh.

NOTES

To make your own pita chips, slice 2-3 pieces of pita into triangles and brush or spray both sides with grape seed or coconut oil. Lightly season with sea salt and garlic powder and toss. Then arrange on a baking sheet in a single layer and toast on each side for 3-5 minutes in a 400 degree F (204 C) oven. This can be done while the chickpeas are baking to save time!

In place of all the individual spices you could also use an equivalent amount of our DIY Shawarma spice blend, which is Middle Eastern inspired.

Nutrition information is a rough estimate.

2. Sheet Pan Shrimp Fajitas

INGREDIENTS

- 1 1/2 pounds of shrimp peeled and deveined

- 1 yellow bell pepper sliced thin

- 1 red bell pepper sliced thin

- 1 orange bell pepper sliced thin

- 1 small red onion sliced thin

- 1 1/2 tablespoons of extra virgin olive oil

- 1 teaspoon of kosher salt

- several turns of freshly ground pepper

- 2 teaspoon of chili powder

- 1/2 teaspoon of garlic powder

- 1/2 teaspoon of onion powder

- 1/2 teaspoon of ground cumin

- 1/2 teaspoon of smoked paprika

- lime

- fresh cilantro for garnish

- tortillas warmed

INSTRUCTIONS

1. Preheat oven to 450 degrees.

2. In a large bowl, combine onion, bell pepper, shrimp, olive oil, salt and pepper and spices.

3. Toss to combine.

4. Spray baking sheet with non stick cooking spray.

5. Spread shrimp, bell peppers and onions on baking sheet.

6. Cook at 450 degrees for about 8 minutes. Then turn oven to broil and cook for additional 2 minutes or until shrimp is cooked through.

7. Squeeze juice from fresh lime over fajita mixture and top with fresh cilantro.

8. Serve in warm tortillas.

Recipe Notes

If preferred, remove shrimp tails prior to cooking for easier serving.

3. Tomato Garlic Basil Chicken

This tomato and basil garlic chicken is a quick, easy, and flavor packed dish that you can have ready on the table in less than 30 minutes.

INGREDIENTS

• 1 lb boneless skinless chicken breasts

• 2 tablespoons olive oil

• 1/2 yellow onion, diced

• 3 garlic cloves, minced

• 14.5 ounce can Italian chopped tomatoes

• one handful fresh basil, about 1 cup loosely packed, loosely packed, cut into ribbons

• 1/4 teaspoon crushed red pepper flakes

• 4 medium zucchini, courgette, spiralized into spaghetti-like noodles

• salt & pepper to taste

INSTRUCTIONS

1. Cover the chicken with plastic wrap and pound each piece to an even thickness all around, about one inch or so in the thickest parts. This will help the chicken cook faster and more evenly. I like to use the bottom of a sauce pan to pound the chicken. Once done, sprinkle each side with a little salt and pepper.

2. Add 1 tablespoons of the olive oil to a large skillet, until warm. Add the chicken and pan fry each side for several minutes until browned.

3. Once the chicken is cooked through and browned remove it from the skillet and set aside on a separate plate for the time.

4. Using the same skillet add the rest of the olive oil and being sautéing the onion until it becomes soft, about 5 minutes. Then add the garlic and sautee for another minute or so. Add the tomatoes and basil to the skillet and season with the salt, pepper, and red pepper flakes.

5. Simmer for about 10 minutes until the sauce thickens and reduces. Make sure to stir occasionally.

6. Add the chicken back to the skillet along with the zoodles to soak in the sauce a few minutes before. serving.

4. Easy One Pan Mediterranean Cod with Fennel, Kale, and Black Olives

INGREDIENTS

• 2 tbsp olive oil

• 1 small onion sliced

• 2 cups sliced fennel

• 3 large cloves garlic chopped

- 1 14.5 ounce can diced tomato

- 1 cup diced fresh tomatoes

- 2 cups shredded kale

- 1/2 cup water

- pinch of crushed red pepper

- 2 tsp fresh oregano or 1/2 tsp dried oregano

- 1 cup oil cured black olives

- 1 lb. cod cut into 4 portions

- 1/8 tsp salt

- 1/4 tsp black pepper

- 1/4 tsp fennel seeds optional

- 1 tsp orange zest

garnish

- fresh oregano fennel fronds, orange zest, olive oil

INSTRUCTIONS

• In a large skillet (ideally with high sides) over medium heat, cook onion, fennel, and garlic in olive oil for 8 minutes, season with salt and pepper (about 1/4 tsp of each).

Add canned diced tomato, fresh tomato, kale, and water. Stir well and cook for 12 minutes.

Add crushed red pepper, fresh oregano, and olives.

• Prepare fish, season with salt, pepper, orange zest and fennel seeds (optional). Nestle fish into kale tomato stewing mixture.

Cover pan and cook for 10 minutes.

• Remove from heat, and finish with fennel fronds, more fresh oregano, more orange zest, and a drizzle of olive oil on top.

• Serve immediately.

NOTES

• This is definitely a complete meal but it is also quite lovely served with a grain on the side, just be sure to pour lots of that yummy sauce over the grain.

5. Healthy Shrimp and "Grits" (Whole30, Keto, Paleo)

INGREDIENTS

For the Shrimp

- 1 pound large shrimp peeled and deveined

- 2-3 tablespoons Cajun seasoning without salt

- salt

- 2 tablespoons ghee or butter

For the Cauliflower "Grits"

- 1 12-ounce bag frozen cauliflower

- 1 large clove garlic, chopped

- 2 tablespoons ghee or butter

- salt, to taste

Equipment

- Food processor

- Cast iron skillet

49

INSTRUCTIONS

1. Fill a medium saucepan with a couple of inches of water and bring to a boil. Place the frozen cauliflower in a steamer basket and top with 1 large clove garlic, chopped. Cover and steam until tender.

2. When tender, place the steamed cauliflower and garlic in the bowl of a food processor and add ghee or butter. Do not get rid of the steaming water! Blitz until almost the desired texture. Add salt and a bit of the steaming water, if desired, and process again until the desired consistency.

3. Meanwhile, make your shrimp. Pat dry and sprinkle very liberally with Cajun seasoning. You want the shrimp to be almost entirely coated, so don't skimp out here! We probably use about 2-3 tablespoons of seasoning. If your Cajun seasoning does not include salt, salt the shrimp now as well.

4. Heat 2 tablespoons ghee or butter in a large skillet, preferably cast-iron, over medium-high heat. Once the skillet is very hot, add the shrimp and cook for a minute or two, or until the bottom side begins turning pink.

Flip the shrimp and cook until the bottom side is turning pink.

When the shrimp are no longer translucent down the middle, where they've been deveined, remove from the skillet immediately.

5. Spoon the cauliflower "grits" into serving bowls and top with half of the shrimp. Pour the ghee and Cajun seasoning "sauce" from the cast-iron skillet over serving bowls. Serve immediately.

6. Minute Garlic Shrimp Zoodles

INGREDIENTS

- 2 medium zucchini

- 3/4 pounds medium shrimp peeled & deveined

- 1 tablespoon olive oil

- Juice and zest of 1 lemon

- 3-4 cloves garlic minced

- Red pepper flakes (optional)

- Salt & pepper to taste

- Chopped fresh parsley

INSTRUCTIONS

1. Spiralize the zucchini on the medium setting. Set aside.

2. Add the olive oil and lemon juice & zest to a skillet on medium heat. Once the pan is warm, add the shrimp. Cook the shrimp for one minute per side.

3. Add the garlic and red pepper flakes. Cook for an additional minute, stirring often.

4. Add the zucchini noodles and stir/toss (e.g. with tongs) constantly for 2-3 minutes until they're slightly cooked and warmed up.

5. Season with salt and pepper and sprinkle with the chopped parlsey. Serve

7.Greek Chicken With Tomato, Olive, And Feta Topping

INGREDIENTS

• 4 boneless, skinless chicken breasts, trimmed and scored on top

• 1/2 cup olive oil (plus a little more for cooking chicken)

• 1/2 cup fresh-squeezed lemon juice (I used my fresh-frozen lemon juice)

- 2 T chopped fresh oregano (or in a pinch, use 1 tsp. dried oregano)

- 2 tsp. finely chopped fresh garlic

- 1 cup chopped grape or cherry tomatoes (I cut them in fourths lengthwise)

- 1/3 cup sliced Kalamata olives (I cut them in fourths lengthwise)

- 1/2 cup crumbled Feta cheese

- salt and fresh-ground black pepper to taste

INSTRUCTIONS

1. Trim any visible fat or undesirable parts from each chicken breast, then score the top with small diagonal cuts that criss-cross, being careful not to cut too far into the chicken so you can still turn them when you cook.

2. Mix together the olive oil, lemon juice, oregano, and minced garlic.

3. Remove 1/4 cup of that mixture and set aside for the topping later.

4. Put scored chicken pieces into a glass baking dish or a Ziploc bag and marinate in the refrigerator at least one hour or as long as all day.

5. When you're ready to cook, take the chicken out of the fridge and let it come to room temperature while you cut up the olives and tomatoes.

6. Gently mix together the cut tomatoes, olives, crumbled Feta and reserved marinade.

7. Heat about 1 tsp. additional olive oil in a large heavy frying pan over medium-high heat. (I used a 12-inch cast-iron skillet (affiliate link) which is great for stovetop browning of meat.)

8. Remove chicken from the marinade and arrange in frying pan so they aren't crowded, scored side down.

9. Cook 3-4 minutes on the top side, or until nicely brown, then turn and cook another 3-4 minutes on the second side. Chicken should feel firm (but not hard) to the touch when it's done.

10. Season chicken to taste with salt and fresh-ground black pepper. (Remember the Feta is salty, so I wouldn't use too much salt.)

11. Arrange chicken on a platter or on individual serving plates and spoon over the tomato, olive, and Feta topping. Serve hot.

8. Ingredient Green Curry

INGREDIENTS

For the Green Curry:

• 12 ounces firm tofu

• a swish of olive oil + a sprinkle of salt

• 2 sweet potatoes, peeled and cubed

• 4 tablespoons green curry paste (I used Thai Kitchen)

• three 14-ounce cans coconut milk

• 3-or-so cups broccoli florets

Optional Extras:

• a handful of chopped fresh cilantro

• a handful of golden raisins

• just a lil fish sauce (trust me!) and brown sugar to taste

INSTRUCTIONS

1. Tofu: Press the tofu with paper towels to remove water. Cut tofu into cubes.

In a large soup pot, heat the olive oil over medium high heat.

Add the tofu, sprinkle with salt, and pan fry for 10-15 minutes, until golden brown. Remove and set aside.

2. Veggies: Add sweet potatoes, coconut milk, and curry paste to the soup pot.

Simmer for 5-10 minutes until potatoes are fork-tender.

Add broccoli and tofu. Simmer for 3-5 minutes until broccoli is bright green.

3. Finishing it off: I like to add a handful of golden raisins and cilantro (I know, I know, lots of levels of weird going on here) and I pinky promise that a quick swish of fish sauce and a sprinkle of brown sugar will take this over the top.

NOTES

Serve over steamy white rice! But hopefully that's obvious.

Swap tofu for another protein if you like chicken, shrimp, etc.

If you need this to be 100% vegan, then you will need to check your curry paste label! Many use shrimp paste or other fish products in the paste itself.

Sometimes I make this with two cans of coconut milk, maybe thinned out with some water, and sometimes with three when I want it thick and creamy. It just depends on how much extra "sauce" I want with it and what texture you want the sauce to be.

IF USING MAE PLOY OR MAESRI BRAND CURRY PASTE, USE LESS!

I love spicy food, but when we tried it with Mae Ploy I just about burned my mouth off. Start with 1 tablespoon and work up from there. However, Thai Kitchen brand is much milder and 4 tablespoons is the right amount for that one.

9. Spaghetti Squash with Asparagus, Ricotta, Lemon, and Thyme

INGREDIENTS

• 1 small spaghetti squash (about 1 1/2 pounds)

• 1 tablespoon olive oil, divided

• 2 cloves garlic, smashed

• 1 pound asparagus

• 3/4 cup ricotta cheese

• 3 tablespoons freshly squeezed lemon juice (from about 1 medium lemon)

• 1 teaspoon finely grated lemon zest

• 1 teaspoon fresh thyme leaves (from 4 to 5 sprigs)

• 1/2 teaspoon kosher salt

• 1/4 teaspoon freshly ground black pepper

• 3 tablespoons

pine nuts, toasted

INSTRUCTIONS

1. Arrange a rack in the middle of the oven and heat to 375°F.

2. Cut the squash in half lengthwise and scrape out the seeds. Brush the cut sides with 1/2 tablespoon of the oil. Place cut-side down on one half of a rimmed baking sheet. Roast for 35 minutes. Meanwhile, trim the woody ends of the asparagus and cut the stalks on a diagonal into 2-inch pieces.

3. Remove the baking sheet with the squash, add the asparagus to the other side, and toss with the remaining 1/2 tablespoon oil. Place a garlic clove beneath each squash half. Return the baking sheet to the oven and roast until the asparagus is tender and starting to char, and the squash is easily pierced with a fork, about 10 minutes.

 Meanwhile, place the ricotta, lemon juice, zest, thyme, salt, and pepper in a large bowl, and stir to combine.

4. Remove the baking sheet from the oven and carefully remove the garlic cloves from beneath the squash. Add to the ricotta and mix well. Add the asparagus to the bowl.

5. When the squash is cool enough to handle but still warm, run a fork through the flesh to separate and remove the

strands from the shell. Add to the ricotta mixture and stir to combine. Divide between plates or transfer to a serving platter and top with the pine nuts.

RECIPE NOTES

Storage: Leftovers can be stored in a covered container in the refrigerator for up to 4 days.

10. Whole30 Fish Taco Bowl with Mango Salsa and Chipotle Aioli (Paleo, Low Carb)

These Whole30 fish taco bowls with mango salsa and chipotle aioli make an absolutely wonderful Whole30 dinner.

Loaded with guacamole, mango salsa, red cabbage slaw, coconut-lime cauliflower rice, and spicy chipotle aioli, I promise this will become your favorite paleo fish recipe or Whole30 fish recipe. Pinky promise!

This Whole30 fish taco bowls recipe is gluten-free, dairy-free, grain-free, and sugar-free.

INGREDIENTS

For the Blackened Fish

- 2 tilapia fillets or cod, or mahi-mahi; about 1 pound

- 1 teaspoon chili powder

- ½ teaspoon smoked paprika

- ½ teaspoon garlic powder

- ½ teaspoon onion powder

- ¼ teaspoon cumin

- ½ teaspoon salt

- ¼ teaspoon pepper

- 1 tablespoon coconut oil

For the Guacamole

- 2 avocados peeled, seeded, and diced

- ¼ cup diced red onion

- 2 tablespoons cilantro chopped

- 1 tablespoon lime juice plus more to taste

- 1 pinch salt plus more to taste

For the Chipotle Aioli

- ¼ cup Whole30-compliant mayonnaise store-bought or make your own

- ¼ cup full-fat coconut milk

- ½ teaspoon garlic powder

- 1 pinch salt plus more to taste

- 1 teaspoon chipotle pepper powder

- 1 squeeze lime juice plus more to taste; approximately 1 tablespoon

For the Mango Salsa

- 1 mango peeled, seeded, and diced

- 1 tablespoon cilantro chopped

- 2 tablespoons red onion chopped

- ½ tablespoon lime juice plus more to taste

- 1 pinch salt plus more to taste

For the Red Cabbage Slaw

- ¼ head red cabbage approximately 2 cups, sliced thin or shaved

- 1 tablespoon lime juice plus more to taste

- 1 teaspoon salt plus more to taste

For the Coconut-Lime Cauliflower Rice

- 1 head cauliflower stems removed, loosely chopped; approximately 3 cups

- 1 cup full-fat coconut milk

- 1 tablespoon lime juice plus more to taste

- 1 pinch salt plus more to taste

INSTRUCTIONS

For the Blackened Fish

1. Combine all spices in a small bowl and rub generously over top and bottom of fish fillets.

2. Heat coconut oil in a medium skillet over medium heat and add fish. Cook approximately 3-4 minutes on each side, or until fish flakes easily. Do not overcook.

For the Guacamole

Combine all ingredients and mash until desired consistency. Add more salt or lime juice to taste.

For the Chipotle Aioli

Combine all ingredients in a food processor and blend until smooth. Taste and add more salt or lime juice to taste.

For the Mango Salsa

Combine all ingredients in a medium bowl. Stir well to distribute ingredients thoroughly.

For the Red Cabbage Slaw

Combine all ingredients in a medium bowl. With your hands, massage lime juice and salt into cabbage to tenderize, until purple juices are released.

For the Coconut-Lime Cauliflower Rice

1. Fit your food processor with the shredding blade or regular blade and feed chopped cauliflower in. Process until cauliflower resembles rice or couscous. Alternately, use pre-riced cauliflower.

2. Add all ingredients to a medium saucepan and place over medium-high heat. Bring to a boil and reduce heat to medium. Cook until liquid is mostly evaporated and cauliflower is tender, about 7-10 minutes. Remove from heat and assemble taco bowls.

Assemble Your Whole30 Fish Taco Bowls

Spoon coconut-lime cauliflower rice into individual serving bowl. Spoon red cabbage slaw next to cauliflower rice. Top with fish fillet, guacamole, then mango salsa. Finally, top with chipotle aioli. Serve immediately.

NOTES

• This recipe uses 1 small red onion and 1 bunch of cilantro total, divided between the mango salsa and the guac.

• You'll need just under one full 14-ounce can of full-fat coconut milk, divided between the cauliflower rice and the chipotle aioli.

• You can combine the guacamole and the mango salsa – just mix all ingredients for both steps in one medium bowl and stir to combine.

To save even more time, you can toss the red cabbage slaw in with the salsa and guac, too.

Follow the directions for the red cabbage slaw first, since massaging the cabbage is important, and then add the ingredients for the guacamole and the mango salsa.

Stir to combine.

• Make it Keto: Skip the mango salsa. I know, I know.

It breaks my heart to say that, but mangoes just aren't keto-friendly. Skipping the salsa will make this Whole30 Fish Taco Bowl roughly 588 calories, 21g total carbs, and 11g net carbs.

11. Turmeric-Ginger Smoothie:

Ingredients:

1 cup almond milk

1 banana

1 tsp turmeric powder

1 tsp grated ginger

1 tbsp chia seeds

1/2 tsp black pepper (increases turmeric absorption)

Ice cubes (optional)

Preparation:

In a blender, combine almond milk, banana, turmeric, ginger, chia seeds, and black pepper.

Blend until smooth and creamy.

Add ice cubes if desired and blend again.

Pour into a glass and enjoy.

12. Quinoa Salad with Avocado and Spinach:

Ingredients:

1 cup cooked quinoa

1 avocado, diced

2 cups fresh spinach

1/4 cup chopped red onion

1/4 cup chopped cucumber

2 tbsp olive oil

1 tbsp lemon juice

Salt and pepper to taste

Preparation:

In a large bowl, combine cooked quinoa, avocado, spinach, red onion, and cucumber.

In a small bowl, whisk together olive oil, lemon juice, salt, and pepper to make the dressing.

Pour the dressing over the quinoa mixture and toss gently to combine.

Serve as a light and refreshing salad.

13. Salmon with Roasted Vegetables:

Ingredients:

2 salmon fillets

2 cups mixed vegetables (such as broccoli, bell peppers, and zucchini)

2 tbsp olive oil

1 tsp dried thyme

Salt and pepper to taste

Preparation:

Preheat the oven to 400°F (200°C).

Place salmon fillets on a baking sheet lined with parchment paper.

Toss mixed vegetables with olive oil, dried thyme, salt, and pepper.

Spread the vegetables around the salmon fillets on the baking sheet.

Roast in the preheated oven for about 15-20 minutes or until salmon is cooked through and vegetables are tender.

14. Lentil and Vegetable Stir-Fry:

Ingredients:

1 cup cooked lentils

2 cups mixed stir-fry vegetables (such as bell peppers, snap peas, carrots)

2 cloves garlic, minced

1 tbsp olive oil

2 tbsp low-sodium soy sauce

1 tsp sesame oil

1 tsp grated ginger

Preparation:

Heat olive oil in a large skillet over medium-high heat.

Add minced garlic and grated ginger, and sauté for about 1minute until fragrant.

Add mixed vegetables and stir-fry for 3-4 minutes until they start to soften.

Stir in cooked lentils, low-sodium soy sauce, and sesame oil. Cook for an additional 2 minutes.

Serve the lentil and vegetable stir-fry over cooked brown rice or quinoa.

15. Roasted Turmeric Cauliflower:

Ingredients:

1 head cauliflower, cut into florets

2 tbsp olive oil

1 tsp turmeric powder

1/2 tsp ground cumin

Salt and pepper to taste

Fresh cilantro leaves for garnish

Preparation:

Preheat the oven to 400°F (200°C).

In a bowl, toss cauliflower florets with olive oil, turmeric, ground cumin, salt, and pepper until well coated.

Spread the coated cauliflower on a baking sheet.

Roast in the preheated oven for about 25-30 minutes, tossing halfway through, until the cauliflower is golden and tender.

Garnish with fresh cilantro leaves before serving.

16. Spinach and Berry Salad with Walnuts:

Ingredients:

2 cups fresh spinach

1/2 cup mixed berries (such as blueberries, strawberries)

1/4 cup chopped walnuts

1/4 cup crumbled feta cheese

Balsamic vinaigrette dressing

Preparation:

In a salad bowl, combine fresh spinach, mixed berries, chopped walnuts, and crumbled feta cheese.

Drizzle with balsamic vinaigrette dressing and toss gently to combine.

Enjoy as a nutrient-packed salad.

17. Sweet Potato and Chickpea Curry:

Ingredients:

2 medium sweet potatoes, peeled and diced

1 can (15 oz) chickpeas, drained and rinsed

1 can (14 oz) diced tomatoes

1 onion, chopped

2 cloves garlic, minced

1 tbsp curry powder

1 tsp ground turmeric

1 tsp ground cumin

1 tsp ground coriander

1 cup vegetable broth

1/2 cup coconut milk

2 tbsp olive oil

Salt and pepper to taste

Fresh cilantro leaves for garnish

Preparation:

In a large pot, heat olive oil over medium heat. Add chopped onion and sauté until translucent.

Add minced garlic, curry powder, ground turmeric, ground cumin, and ground coriander. Cook for 1-2 minutes until fragrant.

Add diced sweet potatoes and chickpeas to the pot, stirring to coat them with the spices.

Pour in diced tomatoes (with their juices), vegetable broth, and coconut milk. Season with salt and pepper.

Bring the mixture to a boil, then reduce the heat to low. Cover and simmer for about 20-25 minutes until the sweet potatoes are tender.

Serve the curry over cooked brown rice or quinoa, and garnish with fresh cilantro leaves.

18. Grilled Chicken and Vegetable Skewers:

Ingredients:

2 boneless, skinless chicken breasts, cut into cubes

1 zucchini, sliced

1 bell pepper, cut into chunks

1 red onion, cut into chunks

2 tbsp olive oil

1 tsp dried oregano

1/2 tsp garlic powder

Salt and pepper to taste

Preparation:

Preheat the grill to medium-high heat.

In a bowl, combine chicken cubes, zucchini slices, bell pepper chunks, and red onion chunks.

Drizzle olive oil over the mixture and sprinkle with dried oregano, garlic powder, salt, and pepper. Toss to coat.

Thread the chicken and vegetable pieces onto skewers, alternating between them.

Grill the skewers for about 10-12 minutes, turning occasionally, until the chicken is cooked through and the vegetables are charred and tender.

19. Turmeric Roasted Vegetables

Ingredients:

2 cups broccoli florets

2 cups cauliflower florets

1 red bell pepper, sliced

1 yellow bell pepper, sliced

1 small red onion, sliced

2 tablespoons olive oil

1 teaspoon turmeric powder

1/2 teaspoon cumin powder

Salt and black pepper to taste

Fresh cilantro leaves for garnish (optional)

Preparation:

Preheat your oven to 400°F (200°C).

In a large mixing bowl, combine all the vegetables.

Drizzle olive oil over the vegetables and sprinkle with turmeric, cumin, salt, and black pepper. Toss to coat evenly.

Spread the vegetables in a single layer on a baking sheet.

Roast in the preheated oven for 20-25 minutes or until they are tender and slightly crispy.

Garnish with fresh cilantro leaves if desired and serve.

20. Salmon with Quinoa and Asparagus

Ingredients:

2 salmon fillets

1 cup quinoa

2 cups water or low-sodium vegetable broth

1 bunch asparagus, trimmed

2 tablespoons olive oil

1 lemon, juiced and zested

1 teaspoon dried dill

Salt and black pepper to taste

Preparation:

Rinse quinoa thoroughly under cold water. In a saucepan, combine quinoa and water or broth. Bring to a boil, then reduce heat, cover, and simmer for 15-20 minutes or until quinoa is cooked and liquid is absorbed.

Season salmon fillets with salt, black pepper, and half of the lemon juice.

Heat olive oil in a skillet over medium-high heat. Add salmon fillets and cook for about 4-5 minutes per side until cooked through.

In a separate pan, sauté asparagus in olive oil until tender, about 5-7 minutes.

Fluff the cooked quinoa with a fork and add lemon zest, the remaining lemon juice, and dried dill. Season with salt and black pepper.

Serve the salmon over a bed of quinoa with the asparagus on the side.

21. Chickpea and Spinach Curry

Ingredients:

2 cups cooked chickpeas

2 cups fresh spinach leaves

1 can (14 oz) diced tomatoes

1 onion, finely chopped

2 cloves garlic, minced

1 tablespoon olive oil

1 tablespoon curry powder

1 teaspoon ground turmeric

1 teaspoon ground cumin

1/2 teaspoon paprika

Salt and black pepper to taste

Preparation:

In a large skillet, heat olive oil over medium heat. Add chopped onions and sauté until translucent, about 3-4 minutes.

Add minced garlic, curry powder, ground turmeric, ground cumin, and paprika. Stir and cook for 1-2 minutes until fragrant.

Pour in the diced tomatoes with their juice and cook for an additional 5 minutes.

Stir in the cooked chickpeas and spinach leaves. Cook until the spinach wilts and the chickpeas are heated through, about 3-5 minutes.

Season with salt and black pepper to taste.

Serve hot, optionally with brown rice or whole-grain bread.

22. Quinoa and Black Bean Salad

Ingredients:

1 cup quinoa

2 cups water or low-sodium vegetable broth

1 can (15 oz) black beans, drained and rinsed

1 cup cherry tomatoes, halved

1 cucumber, diced

1/2 red onion, finely chopped

1/4 cup fresh cilantro, chopped

Juice of 2 limes

2 tablespoons olive oil

1 teaspoon ground cumin

Salt and black pepper to taste

Preparation:

Rinse quinoa thoroughly under cold water. In a saucepan, combine quinoa and water or broth.

Bring to a boil, then reduce heat, cover, and simmer for 15-20 minutes or until quinoa is cooked and liquid is absorbed.

In a large mixing bowl, combine cooked quinoa, black beans, cherry tomatoes, cucumber, red onion, and fresh cilantro.

In a separate bowl, whisk together lime juice, olive oil, ground cumin, salt, and black pepper.

Pour the dressing over the quinoa mixture and toss to combine.

Refrigerate for at least 30 minutes before serving to allow flavors to meld.

23. Grilled Chicken with Sweet Potato and Broccoli

Ingredients:

2 boneless, skinless chicken breasts

2 medium sweet potatoes, peeled and cubed

2 cups broccoli florets

2 tablespoons olive oil

1 teaspoon dried rosemary

1 teaspoon garlic powder

Salt and black pepper to taste

Preparation:

Preheat your grill to medium-high heat.

Season chicken breasts with olive oil, dried rosemary, garlic powder, salt, and black pepper.

Grill chicken for about 6-7 minutes per side or until cooked through.

Toss sweet potato cubes and broccoli florets in olive oil, salt, and black pepper.

Grill the sweet potatoes and broccoli in a grill basket or on aluminum foil for about 10-15 minutes or until tender and slightly charred.

Serve the grilled chicken alongside the sweet potatoes and broccoli.

24. 6. Lentil and Vegetable Soup

Ingredients:

1 cup green or brown lentils, rinsed and drained

1 onion, chopped

2 carrots, diced

2 celery stalks, chopped

2 cloves garlic, minced

6 cups low-sodium vegetable broth

1 can (14 oz) diced tomatoes

1 teaspoon ground turmeric

1 teaspoon ground cumin

1 teaspoon paprika

1 bay leaf

Salt and black pepper to taste

Fresh parsley for garnish

Preparation:

In a large pot, sauté chopped onion, carrots, and celery in a bit of olive oil until softened.

Add minced garlic, ground turmeric, ground cumin, and paprika. Stir and cook for 1-2 minutes until fragrant.

Add lentils, diced tomatoes, vegetable broth, bay leaf, salt, and black pepper.

Bring the soup to a boil, then reduce the heat to low, cover, and simmer for about 25-30 minutes or until the lentils are tender.

Remove the bay leaf and adjust seasoning if needed.

Serve hot, garnished with fresh parsley.

25. Greek Salad with Chickpeas

Ingredients:

2 cups cooked chickpeas

1 cucumber, diced

1 cup cherry tomatoes, halved

1/2 red onion, thinly sliced

1/2 cup Kalamata olives, pitted and halved

1/2 cup crumbled feta cheese

1/4 cup fresh parsley, chopped

2 tablespoons extra-virgin olive oil

2 tablespoons red wine vinegar

1 teaspoon dried oregano

Salt and black pepper to taste

Preparation:

In a large salad bowl, combine cooked chickpeas, diced cucumber, cherry tomatoes, red onion, olives, feta cheese, and chopped parsley.

In a small bowl, whisk together olive oil, red wine vinegar, dried oregano, salt, and black pepper.

Pour the dressing over the salad and toss to combine.

Serve immediately as a refreshing and nutritious salad.

26. Spinach and Berry Smoothie

Ingredients:

2 cups fresh spinach leaves

1 cup mixed berries (blueberries, strawberries, raspberries)

1 banana

1 cup unsweetened almond milk

1 tablespoon chia seeds

1 tablespoon honey or maple syrup (optional)

Ice cubes

Preparation:

In a blender, combine spinach, mixed berries, banana, almond milk, chia seeds, and honey or maple syrup if using.

Blend until smooth and creamy, adding ice cubes to reach your desired consistency.

Pour into glasses and enjoy this nutrient-packed smoothie.

27. Baked Turmeric Chicken

Ingredients:

4 boneless, skinless chicken breasts

2 teaspoons turmeric powder

1 teaspoon ground coriander

1 teaspoon paprika

1/2 teaspoon garlic powder

1/2 teaspoon ground ginger

Juice of 1 lemon

2 tablespoons olive oil

Salt and black pepper to taste

Preparation:

Preheat the oven to 375°F (190°C).

In a small bowl, mix together turmeric powder, ground coriander, paprika, garlic powder, ground ginger, salt, and black pepper.

Rub the spice mixture evenly over the chicken breasts.

In a separate bowl, whisk together lemon juice and olive oil.

Place the chicken breasts in a baking dish and drizzle with the lemon juice and olive oil mixture.

Bake for about 25-30 minutes or until the chicken is cooked through and no longer pink in the center.

Serve with your choice of vegetables or grains.

28. Quinoa Stuffed Bell Peppers

Ingredients:

4 large bell peppers, halved and seeds removed

1 cup quinoa

2 cups water or low-sodium vegetable broth

1 can (15 oz) black beans, drained and rinsed

1 cup corn kernels (fresh, frozen, or canned)

1 cup diced tomatoes

1 teaspoon ground cumin

1/2 teaspoon chili powder

1/2 teaspoon smoked paprika

Salt and black pepper to taste

1 cup shredded cheddar cheese (optional)

Preparation:

Preheat the oven to 375°F (190°C).

Rinse quinoa thoroughly under cold water. In a saucepan, combine quinoa and water or broth. Bring to a boil, then reduce heat, cover, and simmer for 15-20 minutes or until quinoa is cooked and liquid is absorbed.

In a large mixing bowl, combine cooked quinoa, black beans, corn, diced tomatoes, ground cumin, chili powder, smoked paprika, salt, and black pepper.

Stuff the quinoa mixture into the halved bell peppers.

Place the stuffed peppers in a baking dish and cover with aluminum foil.

Bake for about 25-30 minutes. If using cheese, remove the foil, sprinkle shredded cheddar on top, and bake for an additional 5 minutes until the cheese is melted and bubbly.

Serve the stuffed bell peppers as a satisfying meal.

29. Chia Seed Pudding

Ingredients:

1/4 cup chia seeds

1 cup unsweetened almond milk (or any milk of your choice)

1 tablespoon pure maple syrup or honey

1/2 teaspoon vanilla extract

Fresh berries for topping

Preparation:

In a bowl, combine chia seeds, almond milk, maple syrup or honey, and vanilla extract.

Whisk well to ensure the chia seeds are evenly distributed and don't clump together.

Cover the bowl and refrigerate for at least 2 hours or overnight, allowing the chia seeds to absorb the liquid and create a pudding-like consistency.

Stir the chia seed mixture before serving to break up any clumps.

Top with fresh berries and enjoy as a nutritious and satisfying dessert or breakfast.

30. Mediterranean Grilled Vegetable Salad

Ingredients:

2 zucchinis, sliced lengthwise

2 eggplants, sliced lengthwise

1 red bell pepper, quartered

1 yellow bell pepper, quartered

1 red onion, sliced into rounds

1/4 cup extra-virgin olive oil

2 tablespoons balsamic vinegar

2 cloves garlic, minced

1 teaspoon dried oregano

Salt and black pepper to taste

Fresh basil leaves for garnish

Preparation:

Preheat your grill to medium-high heat.

In a bowl, whisk together olive oil, balsamic vinegar, minced garlic, dried oregano, salt, and black pepper to create the marinade.

Brush the marinade over the sliced vegetables, making sure they are well-coated.

Grill the vegetables for about 3-5 minutes per side until they are tender and have grill marks.

Arrange the grilled vegetables on a serving platter.

Garnish with fresh basil leaves and drizzle any remaining marinade over the top.

Serve as a vibrant and flavorful Mediterranean salad.

31. Almond-Crusted Baked Fish

Ingredients:

4 white fish fillets (such as cod or haddock)

1/2 cup almond meal

1/4 cup grated Parmesan cheese

1 teaspoon dried thyme

1 teaspoon lemon zest

Salt and black pepper to taste

2 tablespoons Dijon mustard

1 tablespoon olive oil

Preparation:

Preheat the oven to 400°F (200°C).

In a shallow bowl, combine almond meal, grated Parmesan cheese, dried thyme, lemon zest, salt, and black pepper.

Brush each fish fillet with a thin layer of Dijon mustard.

Press the mustard-coated side of each fillet into the almond mixture, pressing gently to adhere.

Place the coated fillets on a baking sheet lined with parchment paper.

Drizzle olive oil over the fillets.

Bake for about 12-15 minutes or until the fish is cooked through and the almond crust is golden and crispy.

Serve the almond-crusted fish with a side of steamed vegetables or a fresh salad.

32. Roasted Beet and Walnut Salad

Ingredients:

4 medium beets, peeled and diced

1 cup walnuts, roughly chopped

4 cups mixed salad greens (spinach, arugula, lettuce, etc.)

1/2 cup crumbled goat cheese or feta cheese

1/4 cup balsamic vinegar

2 tablespoons extra-virgin olive oil

1 tablespoon honey

Salt and black pepper to taste

Preparation:

Preheat the oven to 400°F (200°C).

Toss diced beets in a bit of olive oil, salt, and black pepper.

Spread the beets on a baking sheet and roast for about 20-25 minutes or until they are tender.

In a dry skillet, toast the chopped walnuts over medium heat until fragrant and lightly golden. Remove from heat and set aside.

In a small bowl, whisk together balsamic vinegar, olive oil, honey, salt, and black pepper to create the dressing.

In a large salad bowl, combine roasted beets, toasted walnuts, mixed salad greens, and crumbled cheese.

Drizzle the dressing over the salad and toss gently to combine.

Serve the vibrant beet and walnut salad as a nutritious and satisfying meal.

33. Oatmeal with Berries and Nuts

Ingredients:

1 cup rolled oats

2 cups water or milk of your choice

1 cup mixed berries (blueberries, strawberries, raspberries)

1/4 cup chopped nuts (almonds, walnuts, pecans)

1 tablespoon chia seeds

1 tablespoon honey or maple syrup (optional)

Preparation:

In a saucepan, bring water or milk to a gentle boil.

Add rolled oats and reduce the heat to low. Simmer, stirring occasionally, until the oats are cooked and the mixture has thickened.

Remove from heat and stir in chia seeds. Let the oatmeal sit for a couple of minutes to thicken further.

Serve the oatmeal in bowls and top with mixed berries, chopped nuts, and a drizzle of honey or maple syrup if desired.

Enjoy this wholesome and filling breakfast option.

34. Cabbage and Apple Slaw

Ingredients:

4 cups shredded green cabbage

2 apples, thinly sliced

1/2 cup shredded carrots

1/4 cup chopped fresh parsley

1/4 cup plain Greek yogurt

2 tablespoons apple cider vinegar

1 tablespoon honey

1 teaspoon Dijon mustard

Salt and black pepper to taste

1/4 cup chopped nuts (walnuts, almonds) for garnish

Preparation:

In a large bowl, combine shredded cabbage, sliced apples, shredded carrots, and chopped parsley.

In a small bowl, whisk together Greek yogurt, apple cider vinegar, honey, Dijon mustard, salt, and black pepper to create the dressing.

Pour the dressing over the cabbage mixture and toss to coat.

Sprinkle chopped nuts on top for added crunch and flavor.

Serve the cabbage and apple slaw as a refreshing and nutritious side dish.

35. Coconut and Mango Chia Parfait

Ingredients:

1/4 cup chia seeds

1 cup coconut milk (canned or carton)

1 teaspoon pure vanilla extract

1 ripe mango, diced

1/4 cup shredded coconut (toasted, optional)

Preparation:

In a bowl, mix chia seeds, coconut milk, and vanilla extract. Stir well to combine.

Cover the bowl and refrigerate for at least 2 hours or overnight, allowing the chia seeds to absorb the liquid and create a pudding-like consistency.

In serving glasses or bowls, layer the chia pudding and diced mango.

If using toasted shredded coconut, sprinkle some over each layer.

Repeat the layers until the glasses are filled.

Serve the coconut and mango chia parfait as a delightful and tropical dessert.

36. Roasted Garlic Hummus

Ingredients:

2 cans (15 oz each) chickpeas, drained and rinsed

1/4 cup tahini

2 tablespoons olive oil

1 head of garlic

Juice of 1 lemon

1 teaspoon ground cumin

Salt and black pepper to taste

Water (as needed for consistency)

Preparation:

Preheat the oven to 400°F (200°C).

Cut the top off the garlic head to expose the cloves. Drizzle with a bit of olive oil and wrap in aluminum foil. Roast for about 30-40 minutes or until the garlic is soft and golden.

In a food processor, combine drained chickpeas, tahini, olive oil, lemon juice, ground cumin, salt, and black pepper.

Squeeze the roasted garlic cloves out of their skins and add them to the food processor.

Blend the mixture until smooth and creamy, adding water as needed to achieve the desired consistency.

Taste and adjust seasonings as necessary.

Serve the roasted garlic hummus with vegetable sticks, whole-grain crackers, or as a spread.

37. Brown Rice and Vegetable Stir-Fry

Ingredients:

2 cups cooked brown rice

1 cup broccoli florets

1 cup sliced bell peppers (assorted colors)

1 cup snap peas or snow peas

1 carrot, thinly sliced

1/2 cup sliced mushrooms

2 cloves garlic, minced

2 tablespoons low-sodium soy sauce

1 tablespoon sesame oil

1 teaspoon grated ginger

1 tablespoon rice vinegar

1 tablespoon honey or maple syrup

Sesame seeds for garnish

Preparation:

In a small bowl, whisk together low-sodium soy sauce, sesame oil, grated ginger, rice vinegar, and honey or maple syrup to create the sauce.

In a large skillet or wok, heat a bit of sesame oil over medium-high heat.

Add minced garlic and sauté for about 30 seconds until fragrant.

Add broccoli florets, bell peppers, snap peas, carrot slices, and mushrooms to the skillet. Stir-fry for 4-5 minutes until the vegetables are tender-crisp.

Add the cooked brown rice to the skillet and pour the sauce over the rice and vegetables.

Stir-fry everything together for an additional 2-3 minutes until well combined and heated through.

Serve the brown rice and vegetable stir-fry hot, garnished with sesame seeds.

38. Berry and Avocado Salad

Ingredients:

4 cups mixed salad greens (spinach, arugula, lettuce, etc.)

1 cup mixed berries (blueberries, strawberries, raspberries)

1 avocado, diced

1/4 cup crumbled feta cheese or goat cheese

1/4 cup chopped nuts (walnuts, almonds)

2 tablespoons balsamic vinegar

2 tablespoons extra-virgin olive oil

1 teaspoon Dijon mustard

Salt and black pepper to taste

Preparation:

In a large salad bowl, combine mixed salad greens, mixed berries, diced avocado, crumbled cheese, and chopped nuts.

In a small bowl, whisk together balsamic vinegar, olive oil, Dijon mustard, salt, and black pepper to create the dressing.

Drizzle the dressing over the salad and toss gently to combine.

Serve the vibrant berry and avocado salad as a nutrient-rich meal.

39. Roasted Brussels Sprouts with Walnuts

Ingredients:

1 pound Brussels sprouts, trimmed and halved

1/2 cup chopped walnuts

2 tablespoons olive oil

2 cloves garlic, minced

1 teaspoon dried thyme

Salt and black pepper to taste

Juice of 1 lemon

Preparation:

Preheat the oven to 400°F (200°C).

In a bowl, toss Brussels sprouts and chopped walnuts with olive oil, minced garlic, dried thyme, salt, and black pepper.

Spread the mixture on a baking sheet in a single layer.

Roast in the preheated oven for about 20-25 minutes or until the Brussels sprouts are golden and crispy on the edges.

Drizzle lemon juice over the roasted Brussels sprouts before serving.

Enjoy as a flavorful and nutritious side dish.

40. Spiced Quinoa and Vegetable Stir-Fry

Ingredients:

1 cup quinoa

2 cups water or low-sodium vegetable broth

1 cup diced bell peppers (assorted colors)

1 cup sliced zucchini

1 cup sliced mushrooms

1 cup chopped spinach

2 cloves garlic, minced

1 tablespoon olive oil

1 teaspoon ground turmeric

1/2 teaspoon ground cumin

1/2 teaspoon smoked paprika

Salt and black pepper to taste

Juice of 1 lime

Fresh cilantro for garnish

Preparation:

Rinse quinoa thoroughly under cold water. In a saucepan, combine quinoa and water or broth. Bring to a boil, then reduce heat, cover, and simmer for 15-20 minutes or until quinoa is cooked and liquid is absorbed.

In a large skillet, heat olive oil over medium heat. Add diced bell peppers, sliced zucchini, and sliced mushrooms. Sauté for about 5-7 minutes until the vegetables are tender.

Add minced garlic, ground turmeric, ground cumin, smoked paprika, salt, and black pepper. Stir and cook for an additional 1-2 minutes until fragrant.

Stir in chopped spinach and cooked quinoa. Cook for a few more minutes until the spinach is wilted and the mixture is heated through.

Squeeze lime juice over the stir-fry before serving.

Garnish with fresh cilantro and serve as a wholesome and flavorful meal.

These recipes offer a diverse range of options for incorporating anti-inflammatory ingredients into your diet while enjoying delicious flavors and satisfying meals. Enjoy!

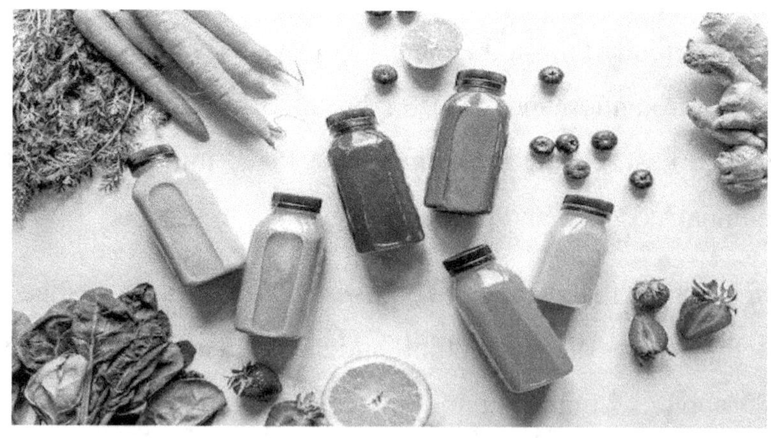

CONCLUSION

An anti-inflammatory diet may help reduce inflammation and improve symptoms of some common health conditions, such as rheumatoid arthritis. There is no single anti-inflammatory diet, but a diet that includes plenty of fresh fruits and vegetables, whole grains, and healthful fats may help manage inflammation.

Anyone who has a chronic health condition that involves inflammation should ask a healthcare professional about the best dietary options for them.

Incorporating an anti-inflammatory diet into your lifestyle can be a transformative journey towards improved health and well-being.

This cookbook offers a diverse array of flavorful recipes carefully crafted to harness the power of anti-inflammatory ingredients.

From nourishing breakfasts to satisfying main courses and delightful desserts, each recipe has been designed to not only tantalize your taste buds but also to support your body's natural healing processes.

By embracing the principles of an anti-inflammatory diet, you are taking a proactive step towards reducing inflammation, enhancing immune function, and promoting overall vitality.

The recipes in this cookbook feature a symphony of colors, textures, and flavors that showcase the abundance of nutrient-rich whole foods at your disposal.

Whether you're seeking to alleviate chronic inflammation or simply make positive dietary choices, these recipes empower you to embark on a culinary adventure that is as nourishing as it is delicious. Embrace this cookbook as a guide to embracing the remarkable benefits of an anti-inflammatory lifestyle, one delectable dish at a time.

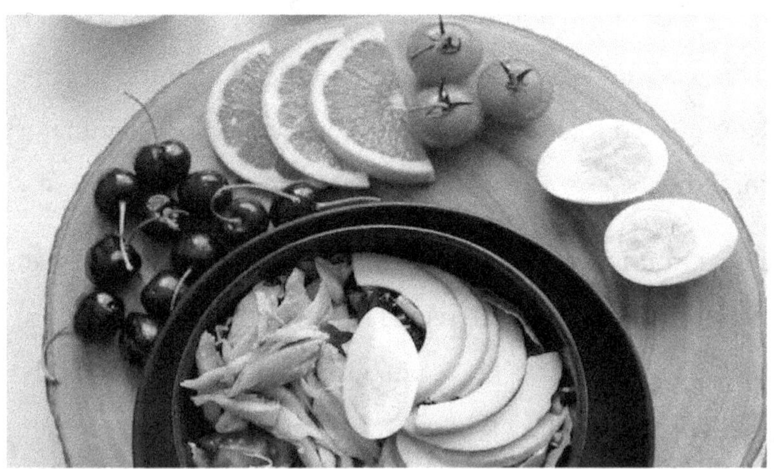